# SLEEP

Ultimate Relief Guide to Overcome Your Sleep
Disorders Effectively

(Roots of Sleep Apnea, Effects on Your Health,
and Cures)

**Penny Scott**

Published by Tomas Edwards

© **Penny Scott**

All Rights Reserved

*Sleep: Ultimate Relief Guide to Overcome Your Sleep Disorders Effectively (Roots of Sleep Apnea, Effects on Your Health, and Cures)*

ISBN 978-1-990268-35-9

**Legal & Disclaimer**

The information contained in this book is not designed to replace or take the place of any form of medicine or professional medical advice. The information in this book has been provided for educational and entertainment purposes only.

The information contained in this book has been compiled from sources deemed reliable, and it is accurate to the best of the Author's knowledge; however, the Author cannot guarantee its accuracy and validity and cannot be held liable for any errors or omissions. Changes are periodically made to this book. You must consult your doctor or· get professional medical advice before using any of the suggested remedies, techniques, or information in this book.

Upon using the information contained in this book, you agree to hold harmless the Author from and against any damages, costs, and expenses, including any legal fees potentially resulting from the application of any of the information provided by this guide. This disclaimer applies to any damages or injury caused by the use and application, whether directly or indirectly, of any advice or information presented, whether for breach of contract, tort, negligence, personal injury, criminal intent, or under any other cause of action.

You agree to accept all risks of using the information presented inside this book. You need to consult a professional medical practitioner in order to ensure you are both able and healthy enough to participate in this program.

# Table of Contents

# Introduction

Life today seems to move faster than it ever has. Every hour is consumed with so many tasks, it's almost as though we never really rest. Even when we lay down in our beds at night, the pace of the world around us intrudes, when we should be resting up for the next round with our fast-paced lives.

If you're reading this, I'm sure you know the drill. Your head hits the pillow and you think, "I'm tired. I can't wait to sleep". And just as that thought crosses your mind, others follow it.

"Did I lock the front door? Did I pay the electricity? What about that doctor's appointment I have to take my mom to? Are the kids really sleeping? I'm not looking forward to that meeting tomorrow!"

Even though we know we're ready to sleep, we can't seem to will ourselves into a state of relaxation that allows us to fall into the kind of sleep we need. Tense and anxious about the demands of our lives, we lay awake at night, counting worries instead of sheep; checking off items on our "to do" lists, instead of becoming one with our pillows.

Then there are the realities of living in the 21st Century that go beyond the pace of our modern lives. The incessant light, for example. Have you ever gone into the wilderness and slept in a tent? Have you ever spent the night in a rural inn, or farmhouse?

If you've had one of these experiences, or something similar, you'll remember how remarkable the darkness was. Almost palpable, it enveloped you as you lay in your sleeping bag, or bed. If you live pretty well anywhere in the world, though, artificial light is a constant reality. Streetlights and the ambient light you find illuminating the night in any place humans live, are ubiquitous.

Then, there's the noise. The world is ever in motion, as cars and trucks whizz down the roads and highways. Even if they're off in the distance, you can still hear them. In major cities, add car alarms and the hum of transformers and other white noise. It's never quiet. It's never dark. You can't turn it off and you can't turn your mind off, either.

How on earth is one to get a decent night's sleep?

The human animal needs, for optimal functioning, Rapid Eye Movement (REM) sleep. This is the kind of sleep typified (as the name suggests) by rapid movement of the eyes under the lids, colorful and vivid dreams and extreme relaxation in the muscles of the body. REM sleep normally accounts for approximately 20% of the total sleep cycle. While we all get it, even if we're suffering from sleep disturbances, it's possible we aren't getting nearly as much as we need due to this problem.

That's what this book is intended to help you with. I want to provide you with a blueprint to move toward sleeping more soundly and, in doing so, feeling amazing! You may think a good night's sleep is something you'll never know, but there are so many techniques and strategies to ensure a peaceful night's sleep, you'll probably be surprised.

Let's explore the world of sleep together, talk about some common challenges and then walk through effective solutions to the problem.

Before we can get to understand how to improve your sleep, it is very important that we ask ourselves this important question; how do you stand to benefit when you get enough sleep? In simple terms; what's in it for you when you get enough sleep? Let's learn more on this in the first chapter.

# Chapter 1: Why Healthy Sleep Is So Important

Sleep is an important part of life. When we are sleeping well it happens without even noticing. When we struggle with getting enough sleep then nothing else seems to matter. It is medically proven that experiencing deep regenerative, and adequate sleep is a vital piece of the overall health of each individual. Many people today will claim that they don't have time to sleep or even that they don't need a lot of sleep in order to function at a high level. This is not true because all people need sleep in order to create the energy tha makes for a tough life.

The number of diseases that can now be associated with inadequate sleep is currently growing. Diabetes, heart disease and obesity related illnesses are all examples of problems resulting form sleep deprivation. It has long been considered standard that each person requires at least eight hours a night to achieve the proper physical recouperation that will allow people to be productive. Some studies have shown that 71% of the population is not getting that amount of minimal sleep required. Many of the problems are a result of choices that people make to either keep working or playing rather than to get to sleep. As this is being written, more and more people are feeling the effects of insomnia. The cost of treating this sleeping ailment has been estimated to cost Americans over $12 billion.

In America there aren't going to be many opportunitites throughout the day for tired people to catch up on their sleep. Napping isn't a practice that is embraced in the American business climate. So people are moving from one tired and less thant productive day to the next. There are things that can be done to help improve the quality of the sleep that you are getting each night. Most of these things don't require any drugs to improve your sleep.

Just common sense practical methods and practices that are virtually guaranteed to allow anyone to get a better night's sleep. A doctor should be consulted before any radical changes are going to take place, especially if the symptoms of your sleep deprivation is leading to any of the following health issues. Heart burn, snoring, stress and chronic pain are symptoms of some serious health issues that will harm your health if not taken seriously.

Taking the inititiative and starting to take action about your sleeping problems might be intimidating at first but looking for help is the best cure for this type of ailment and you will be amazed at how simple the solutions are and the changes that a greater quality of sleep will bring to your life.

In some cases a sleep disorder could be an attempt to tell a person that something is wrong physically or mentally. It is generally believed that those who are healthy will sleep well but if thereis a physical or mental issue then the sleep disorder is ther result. That is one of the reasons that finding the cause and the cure for your sleeping problem is very important. This book will try to help illuminate possible causes of poor sleep and guide people to techniques and theories that will allow for a return to sleep.

If you are wondering if you have a sleep disorder then there are some straightforward symptoms to look for that should be looked for in order to find the solution.

Possible Symptoms of a sleeping disorder.

1. Feeling sleepy and very irritable through the day.

2.Difficulty not falling asleep when sitting and relaxing.

3.Feeling exhausted and falling asleep while driving a vehicle.

4.Concentration is difficult to maintain.

5.Constant appearance of being tired, circles under eyes, etc.

6.Reaction times are slowed noticably.

7.Prone to emotional outbursts which are not typical.

8.Constantly feel like you need more rest each day

9.Feel that caffeine is a requirment to stay awake and functioning.

If any of the above are applying to your life right now then you may have a sleepijng disorder and it might be time to do somethng about it.

## Chapter 2: An Insight Into The Symptoms Of Sleep Apnea

The symptoms of sleep apnea of both types are overlapping and may be hard to distinguish from other illnesses because these are commonly occurring conditions.

Two of these symptoms might seem to be contradictory: hypersomnia and insomnia. Hypersomnia is the excessive sleepiness during the daytime, sometimes taken as laziness, which makes it a stigma. This is why most people refuse to acknowledge their sleepy mood and force themselves into normal function. Insomnia is the inability to stay asleep and it can either prevent you from sleeping or make you wake up during the night multiple times.

Other sleep apnea symptoms include load snoring, which is sometimes due to obstructed airways, morning headaches, episodes of breathing cession witnessed by another person and episodes of waking up frightened, accompanied by short breathing and high heart rate. Waking up with a sore throat for no particular reason or with an over-dried mouth are also symptoms of sleep apnea.

In terms of daily function, sleep apnea leads to attention issues and inability to concentrate. Not getting enough sleep has a huge impact on your productivity as well as on your relationships; sleep apnea can lead to depression and emotional instability. Anger management issues can wreak havoc on relationships and can make you seem an unfit person, all of a sudden. This will decrease your ability to bond with other people and may end in unemployment as well as loneliness.

During the sleep, your body refuels its energy stocks and restores any damage from the daily life, caused by pollution and many other factors we are unaware of and can't avoid. Without sleep, your mental and cognitive state will deteriorate, leading to permanent or partial impairment.

If you experience any of the above symptoms you should check with your doctor. However, none of these symptoms are specific to sleep apnea, so you might need to answer a set of questions to help your doctor diagnose your condition. If you can, it would be good to take your partner with you as he/she can assess your sleep and your snoring level and can signal on specific patterns in it, like a pause in a snoring phase.

Another symptom that is easily overseen is the presence of frequent choking dreams;

if you dream on how someone takes your breath away, in a less romantic way, you might be actually watching a visual SOS from your brain, as you could be actually undergoing an apnea crisis.

Remember these symptoms can also signal a more severe health issue, so do not postpone the visit to your doctor.

# Chapter 3: Relaxation Techniques

It is a normal thing to be worried when you are obviously having sleeping problems. Most of us will resort right away to the use of sleeping pills. Indeed, these pills might be effective but this option doesn't really cure the cause of the problem. In the long run, the body could develop an immune reaction to the quantity of sleeping pills that you are taking. This leads to addiction.

It is scientifically proven that a tense body and mind are precursors to sleeping problems. For this reason, the remedy for it could be as simple as performing relaxation exercises. Again, these exercises will take time to learn and get used to. The rewards are there all right. It might not matter that much but when you are already experiencing chronic insomnia; the comfort that it can provide will mean everything.

Relaxation techniques for purposes of sleep problem remediation and improvement of sleep quality will vary greatly. This is something that would depend on the area of expertise of the person being asked. Tips and techniques are found all over the internet. To make things simple for you, only the most effective techniques have been included on this chapter.

Mind Relaxation Techniques

Thought Filtration – This technique involves the stoppage or removal of thoughts that distract and keep your mind awake. When you find yourself thinking about these types of thoughts, control it and cast it away. Mentally cry out words such as "stop", "don't", or even "away" to clear your mind of these mind distractors.

Purpose Reversal – The more that you worry about not being able to fall asleep, the more it will aggravate your insomnia. Instead of doing this, try to aim to be awake as long as possible. The task could actually fool your body into falling asleep.

Tension Exhalation – This is a breathing technique that many of us are quite familiar with. Breathe deeply and slowly. Visualize your tension being exhaled out for every cycle of breathing.

Float Thought – As the name of the technique implies, you should lie down on your bed and imagine your body to be floating. This is to be done with your eyes closed. Think of your body as a floating feather, an escalator moving in slow motion, or a cloud slowly meeting the ground.

Sleep Counting – You probably have seen this on television and in the movies. Yes, it works but you have to visualize the numbers being written by a calligrapher in a very slow but steady motion.

Vivid Imagery Generation – You should create pictures of anything that would calm your mind. It can be a beach, a garden with flowers, or a perfectly calm snow covered mountain side. The secret here is to be as attentive as possible even to the tiniest detail. Try to involve as many senses as possible in the process. This is one of the most effective ways to get your mind relaxed in preparation for sleep.

Body Relaxation Techniques

Massage –This is an effective way to relax tensed and tired muscles. It will become even more effective if done by a professional or when combined with the use of aromatherapy techniques.

PMR (Progressive Muscle Relaxation) – Slowly tense your muscle and relax it afterwards. Do this for each muscle group in your body. Best results can be achieved if you will start from your toes and work progressively upwards.

Exercise – Light exercise before bedtime releases endorphins within the body. It could induce sleep and make your night rest period really relaxing. Best forms of exercise include yoga and tai-chi.

A relaxed mind and body, when achieved by an individual like you, could make the task of falling asleep almost effortless. Try to use one or two of the techniques mentioned above and see which one would match your actual needs. Now that you have learned how to relax, we shall move on to a very important part of sleep which is dreaming.

# Chapter 4: Stages Of Sleep

First of all, don't think of sleep as a time when your body "shuts down". Think of it as an active physiological process that kicks off as soon as you shut your eyes and go into sub-consciousness. The first thing that happens when you go into sleep is a dip in the metabolism rate. Other than that, all major organs continue to function with no disruption in their working. The intensity with which the organs work depends on the type of sleep you're in.

Remember, taking 10, 1 hour naps with intervals is not same as sleeping for 10 hours straight.

There are two types of sleep, Rapid Eye Movement (REM) sleep and non-REM sleep. Scientists have developed clear links to body issues by studying patients' brain activity through a special machine, EEG.

NREM Sleep

Non-Rapid Eye Movement sleep is a type of sleep that is highlighted by reduction in physiological activity. As the duration of sleep increases, the breathing & heart rate go down while the blood pressure drop. This type consists of four stages.

Stage 1 – this may be thought of as a hybrid stage when your body is make transition from being awake to going asleep. Brain waves start to slow down while there may be muscle contractions in different part of the body.

Stage 2 – this is a period of light sleep and starts off when eye movements come to a halt. Brain waves become slower generally, except for a few infrequent bursts called sleep spindles. The muscles go into relaxation and body temperature drops.

Stages 3 & 4 – together, these stages are called slow wave sleep and are filled with special types of brain waves called delta waves. The blood pressure falls considerably, the temperature even lower while the breathing slows down. The body becomes completely immobile.

The muscles do have their ability to function but due to the absence of eye movement, it is nearly impossible. When people are woken up at this particular stage of their sleep, they may feel tired and disoriented for a couple of minutes before they normalize. It is also at this very stage that many people experience night terrors and sleepwalking.

REM Sleep

This is the second type of sleep which is marked by serious brain activity. Brain waves come in a desynchronized manner that are similar to those generated when a person is awake. Breathing is rapid and changes rate spontaneously while eyes move randomly in all directions. Limb muscles go into a temporary paralyzed state while the heart rate rises. This is the sleep stage in which dreams occur.

By the looks of it, you may think of REM sleep as the villain but striking the right balance between the two types of sleep is very much necessary for a healthy lifestyle.

During a normal sleeping schedule, the body alternates between REM and NREM stages at night. The pattern is predictable through the use of sensors. A complete sleep cycle consists of NREM and REM stages that change position every 90 – 110 minutes. They must alternate at least 4 times in a night or symptoms of sleep deprivation start kicking in during the waking time period.

Adults spend more than half of their total sleeping time in Stage 2 sleep, 20% in REM sleep and the remaining in all the other stages. The amount of time spent in each stage isn't constant and sometimes shows awkward behavior. As we go deep into the night. The REM period increases while the relaxing portion decreases. By morning all sleep is either REM, or non-REM stage 1 & 2.

With that being said, you are now ready to get a solid picture of how much sleep is necessary for keeping the balance intact. Take a look at the following table:

Age   Sleeping Time

**Newborns i.e. 0 - 2 months**  12 - 18 hours

**Infants i.e. 3 - 11 months** 14 - 15 hours

**Toddlers i.e. 1 - 3 years** 12 - 14 hours

**Pre-school children i.e. 3 - 5 years** 11 - 13 hours

**School-age children i.e. 5 - 10 years** 10 - 11 hours

**Teens i.e. 10 - 17 years** 8 - 9 hours

**Adults i.e. 18 +**7 - 9 hours

# Chapter 5: Simple Lifestyle Changes For Mild Apneics

Your risk to developing sleep apnea is increased by several factors. According to studies, gender, weight, age and race are factors that may contribute to your risk. Being related to someone affected by this disorder increases your risk further.

Alcohol use and smoking can put you at risk or worsen sleep apnea. Being a muscle relaxant, alcohol can cause episodes of apnea. Moreover, alcohol use can prolong the duration of sleep apnea episodes.

On the other hand, smokers are 2.5 times more likely to have sleep apnea than non smokers. Cigarette smoking causes the airway tissue, throat and nose to swell. As a result, the air passage is constricted further which contribute to the dangers of sleep apnea.

In the treatment of apnea, patients are advised to make lifestyle changes. This includes quitting smoking and reducing alcohol consumption. In fact, quitting the habit is essential in the successful treatment of apneic smokers. And such lifestyle changes may suffice for mild cases of sleep apnea. With this said, below are some of the simple things you can do on your own to overcome or at least relieve some of the symptoms of sleep apnea.

Lose Weight When Necessary

Like alcohol use and smoking, obesity increases the risk to sleep apnea. While it is true that not all sleep apneics have weight problems, most of them are. According to research, losing weight helps sleep apneics.

By making an effort to lose even just a moderate amount can help significantly with the case of a sleep apneic. Several studies have proven weight loss can either make the symptoms less severe or overcome the disorder altogether.

Limit Alcohol Consumption and Quit Smoking

Smoking and alcohol can have ill effects on one's health. And as mentioned previously, it can worsen the condition of sleep apneics by aggravating its symptoms including breathing pauses and snoring. Someone who smokes or drinks and diagnosed of this disorder should make it a point to either quit or limit alcohol consumption in order to get better in the name of health.

Avoid alcoholic drinks especially at night. As alcohol relaxes the muscles located at the back of the throat, it will only cause more problems with your breathing rhythm.

In addition to alcohol, it is also essential that you avoid caffeinated drinks or taking sedatives such as sleeping pills. These things will interrupt with your normal sleep rhythm further.

Quitting smoking could be a challenge. Before you do, make sure you are properly informed about the possible withdrawal symptoms. Set proper expectations so you can prepare yourself well for the task at hand. But you should also know that doing this is for the better. It will not be easy but doing it for your health makes it worth the effort.

Stick to a Healthy Diet

Studies show that sleep apneics are more likely those who indulge in unhealthy foods. Because apneics are typically sleep deprived, they are likely to have increased cravings specifically for carbohydrates, fat, protein and saturated fatty acids. In which case, they are also at more risk of gaining weight. This starts a vicious cycle. To stop this cycle, people diagnosed of sleep apnea should practice self discipline and plan their diets carefully. As much as possible, it is essential for them to stick to healthy foods.

Eat Moderately

You must eat in moderation. Taking heavy meals must be avoided especially before bedtime. Heavy meals and unhealthy diet tend to cause more sleeping problems turning your condition for the worse.

Keep Your Nasal Passages Open

Nasal allergies can further complicate the disorder. And it will also make getting sleep much more difficult. When such allergies are out of control, a sleep apneic will have much more trouble breathing. And that can be dangerous especially in the case of obstructive sleep apnea.

Items such as saline sprays, nasal dilators, neti pot and breathing strips could help in this regard.

Keep a steady Sleeping Schedule

One of the most crucial steps in dealing with sleep apnea is to arrange a sleeping schedule and sticking to it. Ensuring that you receive enough sleep time every night is essential. A steady sleep schedule may be able to help relieve or reduce the sleep apnea episodes.

# Chapter 6: What Happens When You Don't Sleep

About Sleep Deprivation?

This particular chapter is dedicated to educating you on the perilous risks associated with sleep deprivation. There is a slight chance that you have engaged in some form of voluntary sleep deprivation in order to attend to a work project or a related responsibility.

Do not delude yourself into believing that sleep deprivation promotes productivity. When you deprive yourself of sleep, you are not expediting your progress in learning, work, or any related area. Furthermore, you are certainly not doing your body any generous favors. Every night that you deprive yourself of sleep had tremendous effects on your capacity to function.

This chapter will outline exactly what sleep deprivation is, what it does to you, and what occurs in your body during the process of sleep deprivation. What you are about to read may shock you, especially if you have fallen prey to the detrimental effects of sleep deprivation. However, in the latter portions of the book, you will learn the fundamentals to combating many of the unhealthy habits, behaviors and conditions that give rise to sleep deprivation. However, you can overcome the effects of sleeplessness with the right techniques.

What is Sleep Deprivation?

Sleep deprivation exists in two discrete categories, acute and chronic. It can be defined as a condition in which a subject does not obtain the amount of sleep necessary to support all vital functions in the body. Chronic sleep deprivation can give rise to some horrendous symptoms.

In a nutshell, sleep deprivation can give rise to the following ailments and conditions:

- Malaise

- Muscle aches

- Seizures

- Temper tantrums

- Increased diabetes risk

- Manic episodes

- Increased cortisol levels

- Under eye bags

- Hallucinations

- Sty

- Depression

- Confusion

- Tremors

- Symptoms that mimic ADHD

- Symptoms that mimic psychosis

- Hypertension

- Memory lapse

- Increased in risk for fibromyalgia

- Decreased Cognition

As you read on, these alarming health effects will be discussed in greater depth.

Hopefully, this particular chapter will truly alert you to the debilitating effects that are associated with sleep deprivation.

Causes of Sleep Deprivation

Some forms of sleep deprivation are caused consciously by a subject who wishes to avert sleep in some sense. Many people rely on stimulants, such as energy drinks, tea or coffee, in order to stimulate their minds and work without sleep for extensive periods of time. Therefore, one of the main causes of this condition is voluntary sleep deprivation, in which a subject forces himself/herself to avoid sleep, utilizing stimulants or any other method.

In some cases, sleep deprivation is caused by a more severe issue, one that requires examination by a qualified medical professional. Insomnia is one of the major causes of sleep deprivation, and it afflicts approximately 33% of all adults. It gives rise to a few distinct symptoms, including fatigue and difficulty concentrating.

Another cause of sleep deprivation is mental illness. Certain psychiatric disorders are associated with extended periods of sleeplessness, specifically bipolar disorder, during the manic stage. When an individual with bipolar disorder suffers a manic high, they go for extended periods of time without sleep.

Sleep apnea is one of the major causes of sleeplessness. Essentially, during bouts of sleep apnea, the upper respiratory system collapses and air flow to the lungs is compromised. This decreases the oxygen transmitted to the brain and it affects the quality and duration of sleep.

As you can see, if you are an individual who suffers from voluntary sleep deprivation, then you can use the tools in this book. If you suffer from a medical condition, recommendations will be made later on for more specialized, medical care.

Sleep Deprivation and the Brain

So, what exactly does sleep deprivation do to the brain and just how dangerous is it? Knowing this is especially critical if you wish to lose weight and embark upon a stringent fitness routine. Your ability to succeed on a diet depends on your emotional state, self-discipline and motivation, all of which stem from a healthy, functioning brain.

In a scientific research study conducted in the year 2000, researchers performed brain scans on subjects to measure their performance on simple verbal tasks after period of sleep deprivation. With regard to subjects who were sleep deprived, they displayed more activity in the prefrontal cortex, the region of the brain involved in high cognitive functions. This implies that they were forced to work harder to accomplish simple verbal tasks. Basically, when you lack sleep your brain must work extra hard to compensate.

The human memory is much less efficient in people who suffer from sleep deprivation. How do we know this? The temporal lobe is involved in short term memory tasks. But, it appears that when sleep deprived subjects are given memory tasks, they use another part of the brain instead of the temporal lobe. Whereas, rested individuals tend to use the temporal lobe, thereby achieving better results in memory tasks. This conveys the importance of proper sleep habits.

Basically, when you lose sleep, you cannot fully utilize the temporal lobe, which enables you consolidate memories and engage in active learning. Instead, you have to defer to another region of the brain called the parietal lobe, and this slows down the learning process drastically.

When you deprive yourself of sleep, you actually place your emotional health in a compromising position. Basically, you decrease your brain's capacity to see the larger picture and perceive an event rationally, subjecting you to far more emotional stress. As noted, you emotional health depends on your sleep patterns.

There is a strong correlation between healthy sleep, and serotonin. This implies that without healthy sleep habits, you will produce less serotonin and therefore, be more susceptible to depression. When you reach the deepest stage of sleep, you allow your neurotransmitters to rest, and rejuvenate their initial state of activity and sensitivity. And when you awake, your brain is able to reactivate itself and produce serotonin more efficiently. Therefore, the less you sleep, the more unhappy you will be. Clinical depression can affect your quality of life, as well as your relationships and your capacity to function during the day.

Of course, other psychiatric issues have been associated with sleep deprivation. This next piece of information will truly emphasize the sheer importance of sleep. Extended sleep deprivation has been said to mimic the effects of psychosis, and it can even cause hallucinations and periods of mania. To truly emphasize the gravity of these psychiatric effects, lets break each of these terms down into easy to understand definitions. The first psychiatric issue that were are going to analyze here is psychosis. As noted, if you suffer sleep deprivation, you can experience symptoms that are likened to psychosis.

Psychosis, by definition, is an abnormal state of mind in which an individual experiences dissociation from reality. Individuals who suffer from psychosis or a psychotic state may experience hallucinations, as well as thought disorders, as well as delusions. Other symptoms associated with psychosis include a decreased awareness of social cognition. This, in essence, can affect one's capacity to think rationally and perceive social situations appropriately. When a hallucination occurs, there is a disruption in sensory awareness. This means that an individual can experience kinesthetic, visual or auditory cues that do not exist in the physical realm. Thought disorders and delusions can impact one's perception of reality. As you can see, sleep is absolutely fundamental. And the lack of sleep can mimic the symptoms listed above in extreme situations.

Another interesting term that was used is mania, which is a state of mind that emerges most frequently in bipolar disorder. Unfortunately, this state of mind can arise among individuals who are sleep deprived in some cases. Mania is a highly aroused state of being that sometimes gives rise to impulsive behaviors, such as overspending. Hence, sleeplessness can impair your capacity to function. If you have a weight loss goal, a state of mania can most certainly deter it.

In the next section of this chapter, you will receive in depth information about other harmful effects that are associated with sleep deprivation.

In select cases, severe sleep deprivation can lead to seizures, in which the brain is overstimulated by abnormal neuronal activity. Essentially, when the neurons fire excessively and abnormally, they cause jerking movements.

The brain and mind are undoubtedly interconnected, and one of the most salient influences of sleep deprivation is that which is linked to emotional health. People who are sleep deprived cannot fully regulate their emotional brain centers. This is because when the brain is sleep deprived, other parts of the brain compensate for the underactivation in the emotional centers. The more you sleep, the more the limbic system, or the emotional centers of the brain, can function properly. The less you sleep, the more you will be susceptible to temper tantrums, irritability, and anger. This will affect your level of happiness, as well as your overall quality of life. It is impossible to reach weight loss or fitness goals without emotional health.

Delayed Healing

During your life, you have most likely incurred some type of physical injury, ranging from a very minor injury, to a relatively severe one. Some individuals are afflicted with severe injuries such as burns and deep lacerations. Studies have shown that the less one sleeps, the slower they heal. In order to heal ailments or injuries of any sort, it is always recommended that an individual sleep the recommended number of hours. Sleep has amazing healing abilities that are often underestimated.

Adrenal Fatigue

There is no doubt that several, consecutive, sleepless nights drastically affect one's physical appearance, in more ways than they may have initially expected. For simplicity's sake, let's begin with weight. Why is it that well rested people regulate their weight more effectively? Why is it that well rested dieters accomplish their goals more effortlessly than sleep deprived dieters? The body has a small gland referred to as the adrenal gland. And when the body is sleep deprived, it naturally experiences higher levels of stress because of the impaired ability to process emotion. When this occurs, the adrenal gland suffers fatigue because it too becomes stressed and agonized by your body's state of being. When this happens, it starts to produce something referred to as cortisol, the very steroid hormone that you want to avoid. When this hormone is produced in excessive amounts, it stimulates increase fat production in the body. And when this occurs, your waistline expands, you increase fat storage, and you compromise your fitness goals.

Premature Aging

With regard to aging, sleep deprived individuals do not reap the benefits of glowing, tight, elastic skin. Instead, they tend to develop dry, sagging skin. This is because without sufficient sleep, an individual does not produce as much collagen and elastin as they should. In more simplistic terms, when a sleep deprive person hits 30, they look 35 or older! When a sleep deprived individual reaches 50, they look 65 in some cases! If you are truly serious about avoiding premature aging, then sleep as much as possible, without over-sleeping of course.

Heart Disease and Blood Pressure

The link between longevity and quality sleep is incontrovertible. One of the most resounding risks correlated to sleeplessness is impaired cardiovascular health. Currently, 1 out of every 3 individuals in the United States dies from heart disease. This means that the less you sleep, the more likely you are to become one of the people. Individuals who are sleep deprived are more likely to suffer from the following conditions:

- Heart disease

- Heart failure

- High blood pressure

- Arrhythmia

- Stroke

Obviously, diet has a serious impact on cardiac health. However, sleep is equally as important because a lack of sleep can increase inflammatory proteins in the blood.

Muscle Loss

Proper sleep patterns are critical in the context of muscle building. In fact, sleep deprivation prevents your body from synthesizing hormones imperative for building muscle. When the brain is asleep, the body uses this time in order to heal itself, and to build muscle, as well. When you sleep, your body engages in specific recovery and repair cycles that are crucial for muscle growth. When you are asleep, substantial amounts of growth hormone, as well as melatonin and testosterone, are synthesized. These hormones are critical for cell regeneration, a vital step for muscle growth. When you train in the gym or during exercise, your muscles experience a certain degree of muscle damage. When this occurs, your body depends on sleep in order to recover and build your muscles.

The process of muscle building is referred to as hypertrophy. In order for this to occur, however, your body must build proteins at a faster rate than it breaks them down. Therefore, sleep gives your body a sufficient amount of time to break the proteins down. Once you have awoken after a wonderful night of rest, your body will have absorbed the necessary amount of proteins.

When you are truly serious about muscle growth, protein breakdown is one of the processes that you want to avoid. This is because proteins aid muscle building. You can actually mitigate this process by increasing amino acids levels. If you drink whey protein before bed and get enough sleep, you can inhibit protein process and build muscle in your sleep. If you are sleep deprived, you will not incur all of the benefits that are listed above.

Impaired Hair and Nail Growth

People who are sleep deprived experience impaired nail growth and hair growth, as well. This means that the less you sleep, the more your hair will shed, the shorter your nails will be, and the thinner your hair will be. If you want strong nails, as well as thick, full hair, then get the recommended amount of sleep.

Poor Aesthetics

Sleep deprivation literally affects your physical beauty. The less you sleep, the more visible under eye bags will be. You will also be more susceptible to developing a stye. Therefore, the more you sleep, the more attractive you will look.

## Chapter 7: How To Make Your Bedroom A Relaxing Place To Sleep

Ideally, your whole home should be a place that allows you to unwind. However, most of us know that there will always be the chaos of some sorts surrounding us. A noisy neighbor, a busy road or barking dogs can distract us and cause stress. Having a place to chill and relax is essential and as you drop off you should be in an environment that promotes relaxation.

Here are some great hacks to make your bedroom a haven of relaxation.

1) Choose quality furniture: When you are choosing the furniture for your bedroom pick quality pieces that are comfortable. When you go to a top-class hotel the first thing you notice is the bed and solid wood

furniture. Surrounding yourself with craftsmanship will help you relax. Nobody wants to sleep surrounded by wobbly cheap furniture.

2)Bedding: When you have quality furniture you need to dress it with quality bedding. Choose pillows that will support your head properly, after all, you are going to spend eight hours a day lying on it! Consider how you sleep. If you sleep on your side, you will need a fuller pillow than if you sleep on your back.

Your sheets should be the softest, most luxurious you can afford. Thread count is the measure of threads per inch of bedding. The higher the count, the softer the sheet. Quality sheets will feel better on your skin and will also last longer.

3)Regulate the temperature: Your body temperature drops as you fall asleep.

Having a cooler bedroom will help you fall asleep quicker as it jump-starts the cooling process. The ideal temperature is between 60 and 65 degrees.

4)Mattress: Do you find hotel beds comfier than your own? Chances are your mattress is letting you down. Sagging spots can affect your comfort and sleep quality. The natural life for a mattress is between eight and ten years and replacing it is important.

5)Remove electronics: Do you spend time in bed playing video games or watching TV? Maybe you need to check your social media before you drop off and whenever you wake during the night. Guess what, this is not good for you! Research has shown that removing all electronics from the bedroom can lead to an extra hour of sleep per night. This can be the difference between being tired the next morning and being fully refreshed.

6)Alarm clock: If you have removed all the electronics from your room how will you wake up? We all tend to use our smartphones as a wake-up call, but in reality, a traditional alarm clock is a lot better for our sleep quality. You can get digital models, but they will still glow in the dark. Why not go old school and use an old-fashioned wind-up alarm clock?

7)Decorate your bedroom: Color psychology is not an exact science, but there is a belief that you should choose colors that create a calming effect. If you want to avoid traditional beige and pastel shades, choose a color that creates an effect.

Light purple contributes to restfulness while light brown creates a feeling of stability.

Don't be afraid of patterns, use rugs and throws to add color and interest to your room. Avoid neon colors and clashing patterns to create a feeling of calm.

A study by Travelodge showed that rooms painted blue, silver, yellow or green provided the most restful sleep for their customers.

8)Aromatherapy: Smells can help us relax and encourage sleep. Lavender and vanilla are effective and can also train our body to associate their smell with sleep. Using aromatherapy nightly will condition your body and mind to prepare for sleep.

If you use a diffuser and essential oils, you can become a master at creating the perfect scent to relax with. Here are a couple of blends that can aid you to sleep and relax you completely.

● Lavender, frankincense, and orange. The lavender is calming and relaxing for both physical and emotional balance. Frankincense has been used for thousands of years for medicinal purposes and lifts the spirits and enhances the mood. The orange essential oil will also add to the uplifting properties of the blend and promote relaxation.

● Lavender, lime, and chamomile: Lavender we know what to expect. The lime essential oil is known to support the respiratory system and chamomile helps combat depression.

9)White noise: A constant ambient sound will help eliminate loud noises and annoying background sounds. Anything that produces a constant sound can provide white noise, a fan or humidifier for instance. If you want to stay away from gadgets you can find a soundtrack to play on both Spotify and Pandora.

10) Keep it clean: Remove clutter and lessen stress levels. Your bedroom should have a bed, furniture, a few treasured pictures and accessories and nothing else. All shoes and clothes should be stored away. There should never be a desk or work area in your bedroom, you are there to relax! Now consider your bed. How great is it to snuggle up in clean sheets and sweet-smelling bedding? Keep your bedding crisp and clean and improve your quality of sleep. When you get up in the morning make your bed before you leave for work. Studies showed that people who make their bed in the morning are 20% more likely to sleep well. Your bedroom is your haven, feeling good about it can only help the sleeping process.

Final tip: Sleep and intimacy are the only two purposes your bedroom should have! No work, no TV or gaming, just sleep, and sex! Condition your mind to accept this and you will learn to love your special room and how it makes you feel.

## Chapter 8: Basic Sleep Mechanisms And The Results Of Improper Sleeping Habits

Our bodies have a basic need for sleep. Under normal circumstances, the body alternates between sleep and wakefulness in a 24 hour period. This is known as a circadian rhythm. The sleep part involves two types of sleep, namely non-rapid eye movement sleep (NREM) and rapid eye movement sleep (REM).

NREM sleep is also known as slow wave sleep. During REM sleep you activate the ability to learn and form memories. That is the state in which the skeletal muscles of the body are prevented from moving, which protects us from acting out what we dream. Imagine what you could be capable of doing! Without proper sleep our hormone balance can be disrupted and this may even lead to chronic illness.

To be optimal, proper sleep should not be interrupted, not by thoughts, thirst, bathroom needs or any other bodily discomfort. Let's get down to business. What is a circadian rhythm and what are the effects of sleeping patterns on hormone secretion?

Circadian                           Rhythm
Rhythm is a part of our daily lives. If you look around you, you will realize that most of our social lives revolve around a 24 hour rhythm. We wake up in the morning, go about our daily tasks and at night we go to sleep again. This all happens in 24 hours.

In the past it was assumed that the internal workings of the body could not be influenced by the outside world. Many studies have now shown us that this is simply not how things stand. It has become clear that the internal environment is constantly changing and this is influenced by both internal and external stimuli. This means that things happening in the world around us can influence our inner wellbeing.

Sleep patterns are a good example of this phenomenon as light influences our circadian rhythm and this rhythm in turn influences the way our bodies work. It influences hormone secretion and the release of neurotransmitters which are the basic messengers for the inner workings of our bodies.

The time required for proper recovery varies for every individual, depending on circadian rhythm, age, needs, habits and health issues. But in general, adults need at least 7 to 9 hours of sleep in a 24 hour time period. Teenagers need a little more, close to 10 hours and kids needs vary between 10 to 15 hours, depending of their age. [3][14]

The effects of the sleep-wake cycle on hormone secretion

The body is a complex engine. In my opinion, understanding some of its mechanisms helps us to take actions required to increase happiness, health and efficiency in our lives. This section is a quick 101 on hormones, some of which you will have heard of.

Hormone release is based on cycles. It is controlled by various stimuli. Firstly, hormones are produced and released on a tight shift regulated by a negative feedback mechanism. In other words, when hormone levels rise, the organ stops releasing or even making new hormones. Secondly, some hormones cause other glands to produce or release their substances, and thirdly, the nervous system is also involved in hormone secretion.

Sleep is one external factor that certainly influences hormone secretion and therefore we need to practice healthy sleeping habits. Many hormones are secreted mainly at night while we sleep. These hormones all have very important functions in the body, showing us how important it is for us to get some quality sleep. Some hormones help us to sleep and by sleeping we support the healthy release of other hormones. Let's take a look at some hormones that are affected by our sleeping patterns.

Cortisol
Cortisol is secreted by the adrenal glands and is the hormone that is related to our energy levels. Cortisol levels should be low in the evening and high in the morning.

This is to help us get through the day on high levels of energy and to become tired in the evening. Cortisol secretion is mainly controlled by the circadian rhythm so sleep and recovery play major roles in the actions and secretion of this hormone.

When cortisol secretion goes haywire, with too much stress or lack of sleep for example, the adrenal glands become tired and this leads to metabolic consequences.

Cortisol is normally secreted in the body under either emotional or physical stress. Physical stress can include overworking or illness and emotional stress may come from life changing events and even everyday stressors. Emotional stress can be brought about by the death of a beloved, loss of a job and even something as simple as stressing about finances or work. When this hormone is released the body is prompted to convert amino acids from protein metabolism (in other words, from your muscles) into glucose for energy. Your body is also fooled into thinking that it has to save up some fuel reserves and as a result, fat starts to accumulate around your mid-section. The body then also notifies the thyroid gland to suppress its functions to slow down the metabolism of the body.

To rebalance cortisol response, the body needs to shut down every day. The higher the stress in someone's life, the greater is the need of proper sleep. That is why sleep is vital.

Melatonin

This hormone is probably the best known hormone where sleep is concerned. The concentrations of Melatonin increase and decrease during a 24 hour cycle. The lowest concentrations are around noon and the highest concentrations of the hormone are at night, when it is dark outside. Melatonin is responsible for making us sleepy. As soon as we are exposed to light again, melatonin secretion is stopped and so we stop feeling sleepy. This hormone has a strong reaction to the external stimulus of light.

Melatonin is important for muscle regeneration and to control inflammation in the body. This hormone is also involved in slowing down the process of aging. When sleep is lacking, inflammatory processes are encouraged and muscle regeneration is slowed down.

Growth Hormone (GH), Prolactin and Ghrelin
Growth hormone mainly stimulates bodily cells to divide and grow. GH follows a daily cycle during which the levels are highest when we sleep. Sleep has a very strong influence on growth hormone secretion.

This is also true for prolactin. Together, growth hormone and prolactin burn the midnight oil, literally, as they dig into the fat stores of the body as we sleep. This helps with energy production and to decrease inflammation.

The stomach produces ghrelin which has an appetite stimulating effect on the body. According to certain sleep studies, Ghrelin levels are increased during sleep deprivation. In other words, appetite increases go hand-in-hand with too little sleep. With more sleep, ghrelin levels are lower and it is easier to control food intake. You are then less likely to become overweight.

Thyroid-stimulating Hormone (TSH) and Thyroid                      Hormone
TSH is responsible for helping out the thyroid gland. It supports the normal development of the gland and regulates

the secretion of thyroid hormones. When thyroid levels in the blood become too high TSH secretion is stopped.

Thyroid hormone is made up of thyroxin (T4) and triiodothyronine (T3). The main function of this combined hormone is to regulate the metabolism of the body.

Sleep plays a remarkable role in the secretion of TSH which in turn influences the secretion of thyroid hormones. Too little sleep has dire consequences for the body. When we sleep too little our cortisol levels become imbalanced and through this our adrenal glands are weakened. When this happens the metabolism goes into overdrive by breaking down bodily substances. This will alert the body to slow down its metabolism and the thyroid gland will decrease its function. Hypothyroidism is a disease that results from insufficient thyroid hormone secretion. This may cause tiredness, weight gain, dry hair, facial swelling or puffiness, thinning of eyebrows, pale skin, swelling of the eyelids, and swollen lips.

Hypothyroidism is more and more common these days, but it is certainly not normal. If you think your thyroid is slowing down, I recommend you pay attention to your sleep cycle before considering any other supplementation. Of course, a consultation with your doctor and blood test is also of primary importance.

Leptin and Interleukin-6
Leptin (also called the **satiety hormone**) is released by fat cells in the body after they have taken in glucose. Glucose is stored as fat in the fat cells. Leptin then travels to the central nervous system where it causes a sensation of being full. Another documented effect of leptin is that it stimulates the thyroid gland to perform its

actions. This helps to keep the body nice and warm while you sleep. Studies have proved that leptin levels decrease during periods of sleep deprivation. This means that satiety from food is not reached as soon or definite as it would normally be. Leptin plays a vital role in appetite and weight control. At least two functions are associated with leptin. Firstly, it crosses the blood-brain barrier and binds to receptors in the appetite centre in the brain that regulate brain cells that tell you how much to eat. Secondly, it increases the activity of the sympathetic nervous system that mobilizes fatty tissues to use as energy. Leptin also helps to control inflammation. Excessive inflammation in the body can lead to high blood pressure and heart disease.

Interleukin-6 (IL-6) can also cross the blood brain barrier and has a temperature increasing effect on the body. Another function closely related to this is that it causes the breakdown of fats and muscle tissues. Like Leptin, IL-6 also plays a role in maintaining our immune systems and in controlling inflammation.

Lack of sleep has a negative effect on Leptin and IL-6 levels in the body. This means that insufficient sleep can encourage food craving, inflammation, lead to weight gain and suppress our immune systems.

As you may had discovered, there is a clear connection between sleep patterns and the hormones which are discussed above. It is essential for the normal functioning of our bodies that we get some regular shut-eye. Make sure you do regular blood test to keep track of your hormone's response.

Now that we understand the mechanism of the body and hormones, let's look at the communication between body and brain.

The effect of the sleep-wake cycle on neurotransmitters
Neurotransmitters are the chemical messengers that carry signals between nerve cells in the central and peripheral nervous systems. These chemical messages help our bodies and brains to function properly. Sleep deprivation has dire consequences for neurotransmitter release and affects our cognitive abilities, memory and thinking. I believe it is as important to know about neurotransmitters as it is to understand hormone functions. Let's take a look at some neurotransmitters, their role and how they are affected by sleep.

Gamma amino butyric acid (GABA)
GABA, which is often referred as a 'natural valium-like substance' plays a role in balancing the rhythm of the brain. A shortage of GABA can lead to depression. Studies have indicated that inappropriate sleeping patterns cause negative effects on the way the body uses GABA. This means that if you don't get enough sleep, you are likely to become depressed. Some other functions of GABA include anxiety control and regulation of relaxation and muscle function. It also plays a very important role in sleep regulation.

Serotonin
Serotonin plays an indirect role on the circadian rhythm as it converts to melatonin. Serotonin also regulates emotional responses and changes. An imbalance of serotonin causes depression. Some more functions of serotonin include appetite control and it is involved in

migraine headaches and pain. When we do not get enough sleep we are more susceptible to depression, loss of appetite control and increased sensitivity to pain.

Dopamine
Dopamine plays a very important role in the limbic system. It is involved in the reward system of the body. Our bodies enjoy certain things because of this reward system, like eating good food, having fun and enjoying activities. It is also involved in our ability to stay awake.

Studies show that the circuits, in which dopamine functions in our brains, are changed when we are sleep deprived. Disturbances in its release or inhibition may lead to severe cognitive complications, addictions and even Schizophrenia or Parkinson's Disease.

Studies have proven that if we do not sleep properly the functioning of our neurotransmitters is severely compromised. Even 4 hours of sleep deprivation can cause changes in our brain chemistry. Every hour of sleep that you lose cannot be taken back, so sleep well and let your nerves worry about the rest!

# Chapter 9: The Most Common Types Of Sleep Disorders And Sleeping Problems

To better understand sleep disorders and sleeping problems, here are some of the most common types:

Insomnia

Insomnia is the inability to sleep. This is often linked to other health problems like stress, anxiety, and depression. It can also be caused by the medications you are taking.

Signs and Symptoms

·You have insomnia if you are having difficulty falling asleep or going back to sleep after waking up suddenly during the night.

· You are roused from sleep several times.

· You sleep light.

·Though you are able to sleep a little longer, you

still feel exhausted upon waking up. You cannot sleep without taking sleeping pills and other supplements.

· You are lethargic and sleepy during the day.

Treatment

Doctors have not established the clear causes of insomnia. Nonetheless, a doctor will advise you to be mindful of your sleeping habits. It is important that you learn to relax when it's time for bed. Sometimes, there are a few changes that should be done with regard to your lifestyle in order to overcome insomnia. Hypnotherapy is also a good option to treat insomnia.

Sleep Apnea

This is a very common type of sleep disorder. Sleep apnea occurs when your breathing temporarily stops while you're sleeping. These pauses in your breathing pattern can be caused by the presence of a blockage in your upper airways. The occurrences interrupt your sleep, thus causing you to wake you up several times at night. Most sufferers do not remember these attacks but they feel exhausted during the day. They also tend to be sluggish and turn in poor productivity at work.

This is a serious condition because of its potential life-threatening outcomes.

Signs and Symptoms

Loud and chronic snoring

Choking while asleep

Gasping during sleep

A feeling of exhaustion during the day

Headaches

Shortness of breath

Chest pains upon waking up due to a sleep apnea attack

Treatment

Doctors recommend Continuous Positive Airway Pressure or CPAP treatment for sleep apnea. This is a mask-like tool that gives off a "stream of air" while you are sleeping.

Sleep apnea can also be caused by obesity; thus, losing weight is imperative.

When you lay in bed, make sure that your head is slightly elevated. Sleeping on your side can alleviate mild to moderate sleep apnea.

Snoring

People snore when the flow of air from the mouth or nose to the lungs makes the tissues of the throat vibrate while sleeping; this results in a loud, sometimes raspy noise. When you or your partner make loud snoring noises, it will be very hard to sleep. Snoring can also cause a more serious medical problem like sleep apnea. Hence, simple snoring should not be ignored.

Common Causes

While you are sleeping, your soft palate (the roof of the mouth at the back), your tongue, and your throat relax. If these three relax too much, it can either narrow down or completely block the air passage. So, when you breathe, the soft palate and the uvula (the small tissue hanging from the soft palate) vibrate and cause the sounds.

Treatment

Doctors observe that snoring is more common in men than in women, and in obese or overweight individuals. Thus, their initial recommendation to patients is to lose weight.

If you are smoking, you have to quit right away.

Try sleeping on your side rather than on your back.

Do not drink too much alcohol before going to bed.

Restless Legs Syndrome

Restless Legs Syndrome or RLS is a type of sleep disorder that is characterized by the involuntary movement of the legs and the arms.

Signs and Symptoms

Sensations felt deep within the legs accompanied by a strong urge to move them

Sensations triggered when you are resting and get worse during the night while you are asleep

A feeling of being pinched by pins and needles. Some patients say their legs become too itchy with the immediate urge to scratch them.

Symptoms range from mild to intolerable.

RLS affects both male and female but is more common among women. Symptoms might start to manifest during childhood.

Some of the causes that have been identified are certain chronic illnesses like Parkinson's disease, diabetes, and kidney failure. If you are taking certain medications for anti-nausea and antidepressants, you are likely to develop RLS. Pregnancy is also said to cause RLS, particularly during the last trimester, but the symptoms usually fade away within the first month after giving birth.

Treatment

While there is no known cure for RLS, doctors still recommend a few practical ways to alleviate the symptoms. Massage and movement help ease the uncomfortable leg sensations. Hot baths are also recommended. Heating pads or ice packs can be applied to the legs to ease the symptoms. Medications like pain relievers and anti-seizure drugs may be taken.

Narcolepsy

Narcolepsy is the uncontrollable and excessive sleepiness during the day. This sleeping disorder is caused by the failure of the brain mechanism controlling sleeping and waking to function the way it should. A person suffering from narcolepsy has sudden "sleep attacks" while working or even while in the middle of a conversation. It is a cause for alarm because it can occur anytime, even while you are driving, which can result in a fatal accident.

Signs and Symptoms

Sudden feeling of weakness

A feeling of not being able to control your muscles

Hearing or seeing things when you are feeling sleepy

A feeling of starting to dream before you are even fully asleep

A feeling of being paralyzed or unable to move as you wake up or as you fall asleep

Complications

Narcolepsy can decrease sexual libido. Some sufferers even fall asleep in the middle of intercourse; that's how sudden the attacks can be.

If you are suffering from narcolepsy, you are not supposed to drive on your own because sudden episodes might occur while you're driving and the consequences could be fatal.

Patients with narcolepsy are likely to become overweight due to inactivity and possible binge eating.

Treatment

Although there is no cure for narcolepsy, doctors recommend medications and drastic lifestyle changes to help manage symptoms. Doctors usually prescribe the following:

 Stimulants like modafinil and armodafinil to help patients stay awake

Selective serotonin reuptake inhibitors like fluoxetine and venlafaxine to help alleviate symptoms of sleep paralysis and hallucinations

Antidepressants

Sodium oxybate to help patients have a good night's sleep

Lifestyle changes are also needed:

Learn to stick to a regular sleep-wake schedule every day, even on weekends.

Take short naps during the day. A 20-minute nap would suffice if strategically scheduled during the day.

Quit smoking and drinking alcoholic beverages.

Ensure regular exercise.

Circadian Rhythm Sleep Disorders

Humans all have an internal body clock that is responsible for regulating their 24-hour sleep-wake cycle; this is also referred to as the circadian rhythm. Doctors say that light has a huge influence on your circadian rhythms. As the sun goes up in the morning, the brain immediately signals the body that it is time to wake up. It follows that when it starts to get dark as the night progresses, the brain triggers the release of melatonin, a naturally occurring hormone that promotes sleep.

When this normal rhythm is disrupted, you will feel disoriented, sleepy, and groggy at the most inconvenient times of the day. The circadian rhythm has been associated with other sleep disorders and sleeping problems like shift work sleeping issues and jet lag. Abnormal circadian rhythms have also been proven to contribute to bipolar disorder and depression.

Jet Lag

Jet lag is defined as the temporary disruption in the circadian rhythms when you travel across two different time zones.

Signs and Symptoms

· Fatigue

· Daytime sleepiness

· Stomach problems

· Headache

· Insomnia

Note that the symptoms appear one to two days after flying across two time zones. The longer the flight, the more intense the symptoms become. It has been observed that the symptoms are worst when flying east than when flying west.

Reducing the Symptoms

If you frequently travel because of work, you have to understand that it will take time before your internal body clock resets all by itself. You will feel lethargic and hungry at the most unusual hours. Sleep comes at the most inopportune of times.

There are a few techniques that can help you reset your body clock when you travel. These travels are definitely scheduled, so it is wiser if you begin to gradually adjust your sleeping time at least 3 to 4 days before your actual flight, depending on the time zone of the place you are traveling to. By the time you arrive at your destination, your body clock will have adjusted to the time zone and you can establish some form of normalcy in your sleeping patterns.

If you will be taking long trips, don't immediately go to bed until it is nighttime in the new time zone. It is better if you spend the first two days outdoors so that your body clock gets used to the daylight.

If you will just be staying for a short time, it is advisable that you do not time-shift or wake up and sleep on home time.

Make sure that you drink plenty of liquids to stay hydrated. Minimize intake of alcohol and caffeine because they can cause dehydration which can worsen the symptoms.

Shift Work Sleeping Problems

Shift work sleeping problems occur when your internal clock is out of sync with your work schedule. There are industries that require 24-hour work coverage; hence, there are workers that work on rotating shifts, early morning shifts, and night shifts. Work schedules change from time to time and this can disrupt your body clock.

There are other people who easily adjust to constantly changing shift schedules while there are some who encounter difficulty. Most shift workers are sleep-deprived compared to regular daytime shift workers.

Reducing the Impact

If your work schedules change every month, it would help if you naturally regulate your sleep-wake cycle. There are ways to induce sleep even when you need to sleep during the daytime. If you don't have control over the changing shifts, it is better if you make changes within yourself. Otherwise, you might have to consider transferring to another line of work, preferably one that does not have rotating schedules.

If your company is more lenient in taking requests when changing shifts, you might want to request for a later shift than an earlier shift from your soon to be previous work schedule. People find it easier to adjust forward than backward.

Delayed Phase Disorder

The delayed phase disorder occurs when your biological clock is significantly delayed. When this happens, you sleep and you wake up later than other people. If you have this sleep disorder, it is hard for you to function during normal working hours like working a 9-to-5 job.

This disorder is more than having the desire to stay up late. It is more common among teenagers, and they will actually outgrow it in no time. If you continue to struggle with the disorder, seeking professional help might do the trick.

# Chapter 10: Can I Sleep More On The Weekends?

I had always heard that you could never catch up on your sleep - once you missed it or skipped it, there was no going back. The problem with waiting until the weekends to 'catch up' on your sleep is that it will not undo the damage enough to help. Plus, you mess with your sleep-wake cycle if you wait until the weekend and then spend extra time in bed. Come Sunday night it will be that much harder to go to bed at the right time so you rise early enough on Monday morning to get to work or school.

If you listen to the National Institutes of Health, the 'normal Joe' sleeps less than seven hours per night. With the fast society we live in, six or seven hours of sleep may seem like heaven. But it becomes a disaster recipe for chronic sleep deprivation.

When it comes to performing at your brain and body's peak, there a major difference between the amount of sleep you can squeeze by on and the amount you absolutely need. Just spending an extra sixty minutes or more would enable you to feel better, not just get by. And wouldn't you also love to get more done? Then don't skip on sleep to do those chores - rest and be surprised by how much you can get done when you are rejuvenated.

Although the amount of adult sleep needs vary somewhat from person to person, the majority of healthy adults have to have between seven and a half to nine hours of sleep per night with children and teenagers needing more. And even though some people have come to believe that our sleep needs decrease as we grow older, seniors still require at least seven and a half to eight hours of sleep. Since seniors often have trouble staying asleep at night, they can ease that burden by napping during the day to fill in the rest they need.

Want to know if your at your premium sleep needs? Ask yourself: How do you feel as you move through your day? Are you alert and energetic? Does it last all day? From the moment you rise until you go to bed, that 'feeling' should stay with you.

Researchers at the University of California, San Francisco discovered that some people have a gene that enables them to do well on six hours of sleep a night. This gene, however, is very rare, appearing in less than three percent of the population.

For the other ninety-seven percent of us, six hours doesn't come close to cutting it.

You are sleep deprived if your skimping on your eight hours. And the worse part is that you probably have no idea just how bad off you are. Lack of sleep may also be at the root of many of your health problems.

HOW CAN I BE SLEEP DEPRIVED AND NOT KNOW IT?

Sleep deprivation signs are much more subtle than falling face first into your spaghetti dinner. Also, if you've made a habit of skimping on sleep, you may not even remember what it feels like to be fully alert, wide-awake, and firing on all cylinders. You may think that is natural to get sleepy when you're in a boring meeting, struggling with an afternoon slump, or dozing off after dinner while watching Jeopardy, but the truth is that it's only "normal" if you're sleep deprived.

You may be sleep deprived if:

• Must use alarm clock to wake up

• Repeatedly use the snooze button

• Have a hard time getting out of bed in the morning

• Feel sluggish in the afternoon

• Warm rooms, listening to lectures or meetings make you sleepy

• Driving or heavy meals make you sleepy

• Need to take a nap just to make it through the day

• Fall asleep while watching TV or relaxing in the evening

• Must get extra sleep on weekends

• Within five minutes of going to bed you fall asleep

WHAT ARE THE EFFECTS?

Big deal, so I might be slightly drowsy, you might think. Losing quality sleep has a huge range of negative effects that go way beyond just feeling sleepy. In fact, it's as bad as being drunk. It affects judgment, coordination, and reaction times.

The effects include:

• Fatigue, sluggishness, and lack of motivation

• Anger, irritability and rashness

• Problem-solving and creativity are reduced

• Trouble coping with stress

• Frequent colds and infections; reduced immunity.

• Concentration and memory problems

• Weight gain!

• Motor skills impairment, increased risk of accidents

• Indecisive, can't make decisions

• Increased risk of diabetes, heart disease, and other health problems

DOES THIS SLEEP DEPRIVATION MAKE ME LOOK FAT?

Lack of prime sleep is directly related to over-eating and weight gain. Without quality sleep you crave sugary foods to give you needed energy. Your body has two hormones that regulate your feelings of hunger and fullness. Ghrelin stimulates appetite, while leptin sends signals to the brain when you are full.  But, skimp on the sleep your body requires, your ghrelin levels go up, stimulating your appetite so you want or eat more food than normal, and your leptin levels go down, so you don't feel satisfied and you keep eating. So, the more sleep you lose, the more weight you'll gain from your body craving more food.

SLEEP CYCLES

Sleep has stages.  These stages unfold in a recurring way that can actually be measured.  Not all sleep is beneficial sleep.  From deep sleep to dreaming sleep, they are all essential for your mind, body and spirit.  Each stage of sleep has it's own role in preparing you for your waking hours.

There are two main types of sleep:

Non-REM sleep is three stages of sleep, each deeper than the last.

REM sleep is your most active dreaming. Your eyes move back and forth during this stage, which is why it is called Rapid Eye Movement sleep.

Transition to sleep. This stage lasts about five minutes. Your eyes move slowly under the eyelids, muscle activity slows down, and you are easily awakened.

Light sleep. This is the first stage of true sleep, lasting from ten to twenty-five minutes. Your eye movement stops, heart rate slows, and body temperature decreases.

Deep sleep. You're difficult to awaken, and if you are awakened, you do not adjust immediately and often feel groggy and disoriented for several minutes. In this deepest stage of sleep, your brain waves are extremely slow. Blood flow is directed away from your brain and towards your muscles, restoring physical energy.

REM sleep (Dream sleep)  About seventy to ninety minutes after falling asleep, you enter REM sleep, where dreaming occurs. Your eyes move rapidly, your breathing shallows, and your heart rate and blood pressure increase.  Also during this stage, your arm and leg muscles are paralyzed.

You have an internal clock that runs on a twenty-four hour sleep-wake cycle. You might have heard of this, it's called your biological clock.  It's is also know as our circadian rhythm.  Whatever you call it, it is run by the brain responding to how long you've been awake and the changes between light and dark.  During the night, your body responds to the loss of daylight by producing melatonin, a hormone that makes you sleepy.  During daylight hours, the sun light triggers the brain to stop melatonin production so you can be a bright, happy camper - alert and awake.

Your internal clock can be disrupted by factors such as nightshift work, traveling across time zones, or irregular sleeping patterns—leaving you feeling groggy, disoriented, and sleepy at inconvenient times. The production of melatonin can also be thrown off when you're deprived of sunlight during the day or exposed to too much artificial light at night

Sleep is actually more complicated then you may realize. You're probably thinking that once you fall into bed, you go into a deep sleep that lasts until you wake up in the morning. And that if you wake during the night, to get some water or use the restroom, when you go back to sleep you do so where you left off. Sleep patterns actually resemble a city skyline, which is why some refer to it as sleep architecture.

In fact, you can actually predict your sleep patterns because they move between deep restorative sleep (deep sleep) and more alert stages and dreaming (REM sleep) all through the night. All together they form a complete cycle with each one lasting around ninety minutes. And this REM and non-REM sleep pattern or cycle repeats several times a night - somewhere between four to six times.

As the night crawls by, the amount of time you spend in each cycle or stage of sleep changes. Most deep sleep occurs in the first half of the night while later, your REM sleep stages become longer and alternates with light sleep. Ever notice that, if you are sensitive to waking up in the night, it is actually early in the morning, say three a.m. rather than right after you go to sleep?

# Chapter 11: Signs And Symptoms Of Sleep Apnea And Diagnosis

How do you know that you have sleep apnea if it happens during the time that you are sleeping? Here are some of the signs and symptoms that you should be looking into to signal us to seek help from your physician.

The major sign and symptom of sleep apnea is snoring. However, not all people who snore have sleep apnea. The pauses in breaths while sleeping followed by gasping of air after each pause is another sign of sleep apnea. You may be experiencing it without knowing it because it happens when you are asleep. If you suspect that you have sleep apnea, then you may want to have your sleep partner observe you while you sleep or you may record your sleep pattern.

Here are other signs and symptoms of Sleep Apnea:

·Sore throat or dry throat upon waking up

·Waking up from sleep with choking or gasping feeling

·Sleepiness during the day

·Headaches in the mornings

·Not getting enough sleep

·Lack of energy

·Mood swings

·Forgetfulness

·Changes in libido

·Insomnia

·Difficulty of concentrating

·Irritable

·Depressed

For children, there may be other signs and symptoms which include:

·Bedwetting

·Night terrors

·Excessive perspiration during night time

·Morning headaches

·Irritability

·Failure to grow and gain weight

·More effort used when breathing

If you happen to observe these signs and symptoms, then chances are you may have sleep apnea. However, you need to confirm whether you really have sleep apnea or not by having diagnostic tests done.

Diagnosing Sleep Apnea

Sleep apnea does not need blood samples or invasive procedures to diagnose. There are simple ways that will confirm if you have sleep apnea.

·Self-examination – the first thing that you can do before you go to your physician is to do a self-examination and see if you have the symptoms of sleep apnea. Assess yourself if you have the signs and symptoms mentioned above or ask your partner about your sleeping habits. If you find out that you may have sleep apnea, then seek medical help.

·Medical and Sleep History – before you undergo a sleep test, your doctor may need data about your medical history and some sleep problems in the past. You will also be asked about the medications that you have been taking, about your level of energy throughout the day, how your sleep was, alcohol intake, problems in mental and emotional functioning, instances of heartburn, problems with snoring, and your usual sleeping position. This will give your physician enough data to evaluate your present condition.

·Physical examination – this is where the physician will check if you have the physical factors that may increase your risk of developing sleep apnea. The size of your neck and your weight will be checked. Your doctor will also examine your tonsils and palate.

·In case sleep apnea is not obvious after tests, other conditions that may affect your sleep is taken into consideration as well. This is to assure that you will not be misdiagnosed and would not have to go through unnecessary tests if sleep apnea is not a consideration.

·A sleep study or what is also called as polysomnogram is done to record your physical activities while you sleep. The sleep specialist is the one who will diagnose if you have sleep apnea or another form of sleep disorder.

During a sleep study, you will have to stay at a private room in a hospital or a sleep center. There will be a monitoring device that will be used to record your activities while you sleep. Near your bedroom is an observation room where there will be technicians who will be monitoring your sleep activity.

There will be monitoring devices that will be attached to you. Electrodes will be placed on your scalp and face. These electrodes will send signals to the measuring equipment that will record these activities. There will be belts in the chest area and the abdomen area to measure your breathing. A pulse oximeter will also be used to measure the oxygen in your body.

There are other gadgets that will be used to help diagnose sleep apnea. There is the snore microphone to measure your snoring, the electrocardiogram to measure the activities of the heart, and the nasal airflow sensor to measure the airflow. There is also the electroencephalogram that helps record the brain activity, the electro-oculogram that helps in measuring the eye movements and in determining the stages of sleep you are in, and the electomyelogram that helps monitor the movements of the face and the extremities in REM sleep.

After the data that has been gathered and a sleep analyst has interpreted it, you will be diagnosed if you have sleep apnea or not. If you are diagnosed to have sleep apnea, then treatment should be sought so that you can avoid the complications of untreated sleep apnea.

# Chapter 12: Diagnosis Of Sleep Apnea

The manner in which doctors diagnose sleep apnea depends upon medical and family histories. They will additionally carry out a physical exam. They will study your signs. If they feel that the indications, signs and patterns fit this condition, then you are going to be referred for a sleep study.

Sleep studies are measurements that reveal your sleeping pattern. The outcomes demonstrate how much and how well you sleep. If you have any issues with your sleeping, the studies are going to reveal the results of that.

If you are referred for a sleep study, it is essential that you get one. The study can figure out if you have actually been diagnosed with a sleep disorder, like sleep apnea. Sleep apnea and other sleep disorders can boost your health risk for strokes, hypertension and cardiac arrest.

Physicians who are experienced in reading sleep studies can quickly detect sleep apnea and supply treatment so that you can sleep better during the night. The essential thing is to let your doctor know about any unfavorable sleeping habits you have experienced.

They would include tiredness and chronic drowsiness throughout the day. Additionally, advise your doctor if you have actually had trouble getting to sleep or getting up in the middle of the night and can't return to sleep.

You could be struggling with a sleep disorder that you are unaware of.

Physicians experienced in sleep disorders are going to ask you about your sleep schedule. They are going to additionally ask your members of the family about any chronic snoring that they have actually handled.

Physicians who are experienced with sleep disorders are referred to as sleep specialists. They can quickly identify and supply the treatment for those who are experiencing issues sleeping.

In order to assist the specialists in identifying what's going on, you ought to establish and keep a sleep journal for no more than 2 weeks. This is the start of the sleep study. Here are some questions that you might see in a sleep journal:

- The time you went to sleep the night before

- The time you got up in the morning

- The number of hours you slept the night before

- The number of times you got up throughout the night

- How long did it take you to drop off to sleep the night before

- What medications you took the night before

- If you were you wide awake when you woke up in the morning

- If you were drowsy when you got up in the morning

- The number of drinks with caffeine you had throughout the day

- The number of beverages you had throughout the day

- The time when you drank the alcoholic drinks

- The number of naps you had

- The length of those naps

- If you were really drowsy throughout the day

- If you were a little tired throughout the day

- If you were relatively alert throughout the day

- If you were wide awake throughout the day

Your doctor might additionally inquire about the following:

- Snorting.

- Gasping.

- Headaches in the morning.

If the results of the journal point to:

- Regular naps.

- Waking up more than a couple of times throughout the night.

- Needing more than a half-hour to fall sleep.

- Continuously being drowsy in the daytime.

Physical Examinations To Check For Sleep Apnea.

Throughout the physical examination, your doctor will examine the areas of your throat, nose and mouth. They will be trying to find enlarged or extra tissues. For kids who are diagnosed with sleep apnea, they generally have enlarged tonsils. With them, it does not take much to provide a medical diagnosis aside from an examination and medical history.

For grownups, the doctors try to find an enlarged uvula, which is a piece of tissue that sits and hangs from the middle of the rear of your mouth. They additionally search for a soft palate, which remains in the back of your throat and is referred to as the roof of your mouth in that place.

How Family Members Can Aid To Identify Sleep Apnea.

Due to the fact that many people do not understand that they're struggling with sleep apnea, it is essential that there is somebody that can identify irregularities while you sleep. The individual does not know that their breathing can begin and stop at any time throughout the night. They additionally do not take into account when somebody tells them that they are chronic and loud snorer.

There are things that members of the family can do to assist:

- Letting a member of the family know that they have a chronic case of loud snoring.

- Telling them to consult their doctor.

- In case they are diagnosed with sleep apnea, advising them to follow the directions, consisting of any post-op, follow-up, and treatments.

- Being there for them emotionally. This could be a trying time for them, and they require all of the assistance that they can get.

# Chapter 13: 2 Hormones That Put You To Sleep And How To Produce Them

It doesn't matter what kind of a problem you are having, it is always a better idea if you can find a natural cure than trying to find one that is produced by a pharmaceutical pill. The reason why this is the case is because medical cures tend to attack the symptoms of the problem rather than attacking the problem itself. A good example of this is if you are suffering from insomnia. If you take a sleeping pill that is given to you by the doctor, all that it is really going to do is to put you into an unconscious state. It will not get to the root of the problem that is causing the insomnia, a problem that often has to do with the hormones in the body.

Our bodies are amazingly balanced and whenever we are firstborn, we rarely experience problems with insomnia because the balance in our body allows us to sleep good when we need it. As we get older, however, the environment around us creates problems that we are dealing with tend to throw our bodies out of balance along with making it difficult for us to sleep. Some of the things that tend to get out of balance during these years are the hormones within our body. Here are two hormones that tend to cause us to lose some sleep.

The first of these is serotonin. Although this hormone does not necessarily help you to sleep it does have a lot to do with the mood that you are feeling. Serotonin is a hormone that is usually released whenever we exercise or do something good for our body. It helps us to feel good on the inside and does a lot to relieve the stress within us. If our insomnia is stress related, the hormone serotonin can go a long way in helping us to get a good nights sleep.

The other hormone that we may be lacking is melatonin. This is a hormone that is put out by our body that does many different things but for one, it helps to put us to sleep. Many people take natural forms of melatonin in order to overcome problems such as jetlag and insomnia. If you find that you are suffering from occasional sleeplessness, a little bit of melatonin in the form of a pill may go a long way in helping you to get the sleep that you need.

EATING YOUR WAY FREE FROM INSOMNIA

We experience the ill effects of issues for a variety of reasons. One of the fundamental reasons that we experience issues in our lives, notwithstanding, is because of nature around us. A portion of the things that we need to manage in nature are truly out of our control, for example, contamination. There are things that we subject ourselves to all the time, in any case, that can cause a wide range of issues in our lives. For instance, eating the wrong things can toss our bodies out of adjust and cause issues that range from cerebral pains to sleep deprivation.

That is the reason it is imperative for you to change how you are eating on the off chance that you find that your body is leaving balance. Tragically, many individuals don't understand that they are losing this adjust, they essentially believe that they are managing the issue for reasons unknown at all. The truth is, whether we have some sort of an ailment or an issue in our lives, there is a main driver that should be found. Extremely frequently, the underlying driver of these sorts of issues in our lives is coming specifically from the nourishments that we eat.

A decent case of this is sugar. The majority of us eat to an extreme degree a lot of sugar all the time and trust it or not, it can influence our wellbeing for quite a while after we at first ingest it. Our bodies dump a variety of hormones into our circulatory system because of the ascent of sugar levels in our blood. For instance, the pancreas will instantly respond with a surge of insulin. Albeit many individuals get torpid at whatever point this happens, it can toss you out of adjust to the point where you really wind up with sleep deprivation.

On the off chance that you truly need to have the capacity to dispose of issues, for example, a sleeping disorder, you have to begin eating better. Take fourteen days and completely cut sugar out of your eating routine. You ought to likewise evacuate a large number of alternate things that individuals consider solid, for example, soy and wheat. You would likely be shocked to discover that you won't just be improving night's mull over a predictable premise, your whole mien will be changed. Eat appropriately with a lot of crude foods grown from the ground and you should see a distinction in how you are resting rather rapidly.

SILENCE - THE KEY TO DEEP SLEEP

A standout amongst the most troublesome things that we need to manage all the time is a hard time resting. For a few of us, it turns out to be practically interminable in nature and it influences each part of our life. Not exclusively are we denying ourselves of the rest that we require during the evening and making it hard to get past these extend periods of time, it can likewise make us lazy amid the day and mist our cerebrum. On the off chance that you are having a troublesome time managing everyday life because of not having the capacity to rest around evening time, you may need to hush the circumstance.

I'm not really looking at finding a cure for the a sleeping disorder, I'm looking at getting into a situation that is tranquil. Extremely huge numbers of us need to manage clamor all the time and it comes to the heart of the matter where we may not perceive that it is going on. A decent case of this is nodding off with the TV on. A large number of us will state that we require that commotion out of sight with the end goal for us to have the capacity to rest. What we don't understand, in any case, is that the clamor of the TV is really shielding us from falling into a profound rest. The commotion that is from the TV is regularly only a cover to stow away other clamor that might be going ahead out of sight. In the event that you need to accomplish genuinely profound rest and wake feeling restored, kill the greater part of the commotion that you can from your home.

This can be a genuine test in the event that you have commotion in an indistinguishable room from you are endeavoring to rest, for example, on the off chance that some individual is wheezing. The main genuine path for you to get around this is to wear some sort of earplug or headset. You may be astonished to discover that putting a few earplugs in on a daily premise will enable you to rest without awakening to intermittently. On the off chance that you do this, ensure you have a reinforcement alert set which will have the capacity to be heard, even with your earplugs in.

It might take a tad bit of work on your part with a specific end goal to find what commotions should be expelled from your family unit. It will all be justified regardless of the exertion, be that as it may, at whatever point you at long last get the great evenings rest that you require.

# Chapter 14: The Underlying Causes Of Insomnia And Most Sleep Disorders

The information about the symptoms that come with various sleep disorders, which was discussed on the previous chapter should prepare you for this one – a discussion about the root cause of the problem.

Insomnia Causes and Triggers

It's best to begin with the most common condition– insomnia. You'd be surprised to know that insomnia is among the most complex concerns as well.

Bad Habits

For some people, that medical condition arises due to bad habits. For starters, drinking coffee hours before bedtime is not a good idea. Eating too much during dinner might also trigger problems with sleeping. Regularly sleeping in a less-than-suitable environment could also lead to insomnia. To be a bit more specific, if you fall asleep while the lights are on or when there's still loud music coming from the television, you might end up waking in the morning feeling exhausted. Norte that deep slumber is necessary to feel completely refreshed, and distractions and interruptions will prevent you from falling into a deep sleep.

Underlying Conditions

Bad habits are not the only reasons why insomnia manifests. The condition could also be triggered by certain health problems. For example, those suffering from arthritis often find it difficult to rest at night. Episodes of heartburn also prevent people from falling asleep. Simply put, any health concern that causes considerable pain is capable of inducing insomnia.

Medication

Sometimes though, substances that are supposed to take away the pain make the sleeping disorder appear. This isn't about sedatives though. This is about antidepressants and anxiety medications (which actually fight pain, although only the kind that affects a person's psychological and emotional facets). Those pills usually have insomnia listed under their side effects.

Stress

Not having inner peace (during bedtime) also brings sleeplessness. So, it'd really be hard to stay away from insomnia if you're considerably worried about something. Past events that made a significant impact in your life (not the positive kind, of course) might also deprive you of sleep, especially if you still haven't overcome the pain that those instances brought you.

Physiology

Some biological processes are associated with sleep disorders. Pregnancy, for example, could bring insomnia. What's the link between the two? Those carrying a child experience changes in their hormones, which in turn creates hot flashes. Hot flashes can be extremely uncomfortable and might cause frequent sleep interruptions or prevent sleep altogether. It's the same with women going through menopause. Hot flashes during pregnancy and throughout menopause are essentially the same because they are both caused by shifts in hormone levels, so it's not that surprising that ladies who are going through menopause also suffer from sleepless nights.

Susceptibility to Apnea

Now that the many possible roots of insomnia have been discussed, it's time to move on to the causes of sleep apnea.

Being overweight is one of the most common causes of the condition. Having excess amounts of fat in the body could lead to blocked passages. The central airway, which includes the nose, the throat, and the windpipe, isn't an exception.

Brain problems could also be the cause. Since the brain essentially controls everything, even processes that are considered involuntary, it could affect breathing. In other words, it can completely shut down the entire respiratory system if it sends the wrong signals (or if it did not send any signal at all).

## Causes of Restless-Legs Syndrome

The restless-leg syndrome on the other hand, is not only associated with the brain; it is also linked with the nerves.

## Nerve Damage

That's why those who have been injured and have suffered from peripheral-nerve damage experience unintentional twitching. You have to remember though, that injuries aren't the only reason why the nervous system ends up failing.

## Underlying Conditions

Any medical condition that has a detrimental impact on the brain and nerves could eventually cause leg jerkiness. People who are suffering from kidney failure for example, usually go through episodes of leg twitching. In a similar sense, the ones who are affected by either anemia or diabetes also wind up having random-leg-movement issues.

Other Triggers

The syndrome could also be triggered by certain drugs as well as pregnancy. Those risk factors make this sleep problem slightly similar to the much more common insomnia.

The Root Cause of Rarer Sleep Disorders

Science may have come a long way, but a lot of things are yet to be discovered when it comes to sleep problems. Narcolepsy, for example, remains "unmapped", which simply means that healthcare professionals aren't exactly sure how and why it occurs.

Like narcolepsy, sleepwalking isn't completely understood by science. At the very least though, scientists hypothesize that the condition stems from a mistake in sleep-arousal switching. In much simpler terms, those who sleepwalk fail to properly transition from deep sleep into being awake, making them temporarily stuck in a state just between slumber and consciousness.

# Chapter 15: Insomnia Diagnosis

A number of methods are used by doctors and health care experts to diagnose insomnia as well as determine the unique symptoms of individuals. Some of the methods used for diagnosing insomnia can be done at home while others call for an appointment at a doctor's clinic.

Various tools are used to diagnose and quantify the symptoms of insomnia. Some of these tools involve being submitted to blood tests; being asked questions by the doctor regarding sleep habits/patterns; filling out questionnaires; or doing an overnight sleep for study or observation.

Doctors and health care experts make use of diagnosis measures that help them determine the severity of your insomnia.

These include a sleep log, sleep inventory, blood tests and sleep study.

A sleep log is similar to a diary, which keeps a record of details regarding your sleep. Details include the time you go to sleep and the time you wake up. A sleep log helps your doctor discern the cause of your insomnia.

A sleep inventory is a type of questionnaire with extensive inquiries regarding your personal health, sleep patterns and medical history.

Blood tests are usually performed to determine if your insomnia is caused by other medical conditions or underlying illnesses that can inhibit you from having a good sleep.

A sleep study is usually suggested to people who have insomnia in order to acquire information about their nighttime sleeping patterns. You will be asked to do a polysomnography or overnight sleep in a lab that is set up with a relaxing bed. During the sleep study, you will be submitted to an EEG wherein your stages of sleep are monitored. A sleep study measures your heart patterns, body movements, oxygen levels and breathing patterns.

If your sleeping problem has already become a pattern, it is advisable to seek help. You may start by consulting with your primary care doctor who is proficient in sleep disorders. You may be referred to a doctor who is a specialist in sleep medicine for further tests.

Medical Treatments for Insomnia (Sleeping Tablets/Sleep Aids)

Sleeping tablets or sleep aids are medications that help people with insomnia get better sleep They are considered hypnotics and usually taken to help ease symptoms of short-term insomnia; reduce very severe symptoms of insomnia; and if non-medical treatments fail to take effect.

On the other hand, doctors and health care experts are often hesitant to suggest sleeping tablets or sleep aids to their patients. As much as sleeping tablets can relieve insomnia symptoms, they cannot treat the cause of insomnia.

Sleeping tablets or sleep aids are unable to take effect in people with long-term insomnia. In general, doctors would refer these people to a psychologist or sleep medicine specialist to carry out other treatment methods.

In cases when you are prescribed with sleeping tablets, your doctor is likely to give you only the smallest dose possible at the shortest time, usually less than a week. Otherwise, if your insomnia is severe, your doctor is likely to prescribe taking sleeping tablets 2 or 3 times a week instead of every night.

Sleeping tablets or sleep aids can also cause side effects depending on the type, dose and reaction of an individual's system. They can result to daytime drowsiness or a feeling of hangover. As such, it is advisable to take sleeping tablets or sleep aids during the night, prior to going to bed.

In some cases, specifically in older people, the feeling of hangover can last until the next day. Thus, it is advised to be cautious if you will be driving the next day or doing activities that call for dynamic reflexes.

## Factors to Consider When Taking Sleeping Tablets or Sleep Aids

More often than not, people with insomnia find it helpful to take sleeping tablets or sleep aids as support for falling asleep, staying asleep during the night or improving the quality of sleep. On the other hand, there are a few things to consider when taking sleeping tablets or sleep aids.

1. Sleeping tablets or sleep aids may be helpful only after trying natural or non-medical treatments yet insomnia persists and continues to disrupt your daily activities.

2. A specific sleeping tablet may be indicated after your doctor has discerned the cause of your insomnia. As such, you should not just take one at your own will.

3. Sleeping tablets or sleep aids are not replacements for healthy, natural sleep habits. The primary cure for insomnia is developing good sleep practices. If your insomnia is long-standing, it is best to still use natural or non-medical treatments or a combination of non-medical treatments and sleeping tablets.

4. If you have short-term insomnia, sleeping tablets may help. If the cause of your sleep difficulty is just a temporary event such as a jet lag, it is safe to take sleep aids. However, if your sleep difficulty persists for more than 3 times in a week, you should consult your doctor and stop taking sleeping tablets.

5. Prior to taking sleeping tablets or sleep aids, discuss with your doctor if you notice health or psychological consequences due to difficulty in sleeping.

Some sleeping tablets or sleep aids are accessible only through prescription. This is because they can be addictive and may result to more serious problems if the type, plan and dose are inappropriate for your insomnia case.

Types of Sleeping Tablets or Sleep Aids

Benzodiazepines

These are medications for insomnia that serve as tranquilizers capable of promoting relaxation, sleep and calmness and reducing anxiety. Benzodiazepines are usually prescribed to people with severe insomnia or extreme distress due to insomnia.

The most common side effect of benzodiazepines is sleepiness. In addition, it can lead to addiction or dependency, which is why doctors recommend them for short-term effects.

Z Medicines

These medications are short-acting medicines that work in the same way as benzodiazepines. They are considered the newer type of insomnia medication. They include zolpidem, zaleplon, and zoplicone.

Zolpiden is a short-term medication for debilitating insomnia, which is usually prescribed at the lowest possible dose and taken for no more than 4 weeks. Some of its common side effects include headaches, diarrhea, tiredness, sleep problems, dizziness, vomiting/nausea and stomach pains. Its less common side effects include double vision and lack of concentration.

Zaleplon is a licensed medication for treating people who have difficulty going to sleep. It is usually prescribed at the lowest possible dose and only taken for no more than 2 weeks. Some of the side effects of Zaleplon include sleepiness, dysmenorrhea or painful periods in women, memory problems and paraesthesia or pins and needles. Less common side effects of Zaleplon include lack of coordination and balance, changes in sense of smell, hallucinations, apathy or lack of interest, problems in concentration and dizziness.

**Zopiclone** is also a licensed medication for insomnia specifically for individuals who have trouble falling asleep, being awoken during the night, and debilitating insomnia. It is also taken at the lowest possible dose and taken no more than 4 weeks. The common side effects of zopiclone include sleepiness, dry mouth, and metallic taste. Less common side effects of this medication are drowsiness, headaches, vomiting, dizziness and nausea.

Z medicines may also lead to psychiatric reactions including agitation, delusion, anger, aggressiveness, irritability, hallucinations and nightmares. Once you experience one or more of these reactions, stop taking these medications and consult your doctor as soon as possible.

Antidepressants

Antidepressants are usually prescribed to people with insomnia specifically if they have a history of depression. One of the most common antidepressants used for treating insomnia include melatonin.

Medications that contain melatonin have shown relieving effects against the symptoms of insomnia. Melatonin helps in regulating the sleep cycle referred to as the circadian rhythm given that it is a naturally-occurring hormone.

Circadin is the most popular medication that contains melatonin. It is licensed for use in insomnia and available only on prescription for individuals who are 55 years old and above. It is specifically used for treating insomnia on a short-term basis of no more than 3 weeks. If you have a liver or kidney disease, it is not recommended to take Circadin for treating insomnia.

Some of the side effects of Circadin include dizziness, constipation, weight gain, irritability, migraine and stomach pain.

Alternative Medicines

There are several alternative medications for people who have trouble going to sleep or staying asleep during the night. On the other hand, these medications do not pass through safety tests as other types of medications. As such, their efficiency and side effects are not determined or understood.

# Chapter 16: Ambiance Is Everything

Creating an environment that promotes sleep is very important if you want quality in the kind of sleep you get. It is not enough that you have a fluffy bed, nice pillows, and a warm blanket. There are many things in the bedroom that can, and will affect sleep. So, look around and check if you have things in your bedroom that will affect your sleep in a positive way.

LIGHT

Artificial light (blue in hue) should be removed from the room. This kind of light is associated with waking activities in our brain. When we see it, we are not only reminded of these activities, but the light itself keeps our mind alert.

Instead of the artificial blue light, choose a pastel yellow light with a warm hue. You can also adjust your ordinary lights, like dimming them, for this, too, will send signals to your brain. Once your brain sees dim lights, it will produce the hormone melatonin—melatonin is the hormone that generates sleep—so, as you wind down, dim the lights and turn off all electronic devices that emit an artificial blue light.

SOUND

Noise is not the only sound that can keep you awake at night. Irritating sounds like a dripping faucet, coughing, barking dogs, fighting cats, and other noises that are just jarring can keep you awake.

To neutralize these sounds you can try to cover it with something soothing. Many people use nature noises, beautiful classical music, the sound of the ocean crashing, or Gregorian chants to lull them to sleep. Some people like folk music, or soft acoustic songs that have light, positive, lyrics. Many find instrumental music that feature only one instrument (piano or guitar) works better at easing them to sleep. Find that one sound that makes you feel relaxed and use it to dull out all the other noises outside your room

Of course, this is not recommended if you need to listen in on the noise, i.e. parents with infants in another room. For these situations, one recommendation is to bring the baby in. This way, you don't need to strain your ear too much listening to a baby monitor because the baby is closer to you.

TEMPERATURE

Keep the temperature in your room between 60 - 70 degrees Fahrenheit (15 - 20 degrees Celsius). Keeping the room cool prevents you from waking up constantly throughout the night covered in sweat. Make sure though that it doesn't dip any lower than 60 or go any higher than 70. Any extreme changes in temperature will affect the quality and quantity of your sleep.

BED, PILLOWS, AND BLANKETS

Sometimes, the reason why we find it hard to sleep is because there are certain things in our own bed that make us sneeze, itch, and just overall annoy and keep us awake. You have to check if the mattress has bed bugs, dust, mold, mite droppings and other things that trigger allergies. One thing you can do to ensure that your sleep is not bothered by these pests is to air-tighten your mattress, and use dust proof covers. Also, change pillow covers and blankets as often as you can and make sure to use hypo-allergenic laundry soap and fabric conditioners if you are super sensitive.

# Chapter 17: Diagnosing Sleep Apnea

Sleep Apnea as a disease is easy to diagnose even at home. But you cannot be sure that the symptoms which you are experiencing are associated with Sleep Apnea. One of the most alarming symptoms is waking up at night, snoring, and being restless throughout the day. But that is not enough to start medication or treatment yourself. You need to be sure and take a doctor's advice at the first sign. You will have to undergo a few tests at the doctors, and here we will talk about those tests along with some self-help tests to help you figure it out.

**Sleep Diary:** Let's start with something simple. A sleep diary is something that your doctor may advise you to maintain after the first visit. Although there are tests to be sure whether or not you are suffering from such a disease. A sleep diary is basically a daily account that you will have to maintain. It will include information like when do you go to sleep, how many times and at what time did you wake up in the night, and at what time you woke up in the morning. A doctor will look for patterns within the information you will note down in the diary. Two weeks is the typical time limit for which you will have to maintain your diary.

**Polysomnogram** **or** **Polysomnography:** This is a sleep study that is done with the help of machines and here you will have to stay under the study for the whole night. What happens is that when you are asleep, there will be several pieces of equipment attached to monitor your heart and lungs. Other than this, your brain activity will also be monitored. Further, the arm and leg movement, breathing patterns, and blood oxygen levels are also taken into account. The type of study can vary from full night to split-night. But the results are what matter here.

These machines will send data and signals to the monitor, which will be observed by the doctors and technicians. In the split night study, if you are diagnosed with obstructive Sleep Apnea, at that moment, you will be given CPAP for the second half of the night.

A Few Other Sleep Tests to Help Clear the Picture:

**Electroencephalogram**: This is a small test conducted to record brain activity. Basically, the EEG is undertaken to identify the electrical activity of the brain.

**Electromyogram:** This test helps to record and observe the muscular movement when a person is asleep. Activities such as teeth grinding, face twitches, and other kinds of movements are recorded.

**Electro-oculogram:** Popularly called EOG, this test is conducted to observe and record the eye movements when the patient is asleep. The benefit of this test is that it can help the doctor identify the stage of sleep.

**Electrocardiogram:** Heart rate and heart rhythm are also observed to help diagnose Sleep Apnea. And this is done with an ECG.

**Sensors and Microphone:** There is a nasal airflow sensor attached to or nearby to the nose. This will record the airflow. There is also a snore microphone attached nearby that will record the sound emitted by your snoring.

Can I Self-Diagnose Sleep Apnea?

Self Diagnosing Sleep Apnea is easy and can be done at home with the help of a few tests. Before that, you can also look after your symptoms and signs that hint towards the presence of Sleep Apnea. Other than this, there are a couple of tests that you can take at home. These are:

**Epworth Sleepiness Test:** This test is taken in a question-answer form. It is a scale that measures the sleepiness intensity during the daytime. And this scale is not just helpful for diagnosing Sleep Apnea but also various sleep disorders. There are 8 questions in this test, and the responses are recorded on a 4-point scale. The primary motive of the test is to measure the probability of sleep during the daytime.

**Berlin Questionnaire:** This is a dedicated Sleep Apnea diagnosing questionnaire. And with this test, the subjects can not only identify whether or not they have Sleep Apnea but also determine its category and risk factor. At the end of the test, your total points will decide the risk level of Sleep Apnea.

Diagnosing Sleep Apnea is not very difficult for the doctors or even for the patients themselves. Even the most basic habits in your daily life can hint at the arrival of this condition. Symptoms like snoring, fatigue, sleepiness, and such other daytime conditions are enough to tell you that there is something wrong with your body. But it is always suggested to take advice from a doctor so that you can get an exact idea about the intensity, category, type, and stage of Sleep Apnea. Even though there are two major types of Sleep Apnea and out of them, OSA has the highest number of cases.

Complications Caused Due to Sleep Apnea

Always remember that the human body is a complex machine where every body part is connected to each other. In that case, Sleep Apnea has multifaceted effects on the whole body.

Almost all the causes that you have read above, which can cause Sleep Apnea are also the complications of suffering Sleep Apnea.

-**Depression:** Depression is indeed a cause for Sleep Apnea, but a person who is suffering from Sleep Apnea can also develop depression. The connection between a lack of sleep and depression is stronger than the association between the inability to sleep or waking up at night and depression. It has also been found that around **46% of Sleep Apnea patients** are suffering from Obstructive Sleep Apnea Syndrome (OSAS).

-**Memory Loss:** Sleep is akin to rejuvenating every system in the body only to get it ready for the next day. This means that sleep is essential if you want to be energized, focused, and attentive for the next day. In this scenario, an inability to sleep well at night can lead to memory loss because the brain does not get enough rest.

-**Weakens Immune System:** A disturbed sleep can also weaken your immune system because the body is not able to rejuvenate well in the night.

-**High Blood Pressure (BP):** Because the blood oxygen levels undergo sudden changes in Sleep Apnea, if left untreated, this can develop into a bigger problem of high BP and hypertension. This happens because when the brain finds that the levels of oxygen are falling in the blood, it demands more oxygen. Due to this, the higher demand for blood increases the pressure leading to high BP. If left untreated, high BP can also develop into a stroke or heart disease.

-**Liver Issues:** There is evidence that obstructive Sleep Apnea is related to liver damage. Majorly, people suffering from Sleep Apnea can develop Nonalcoholic fatty liver disease (NAFLD). It can also lead to liver failure. Earlier it was believed that NAFLD was associated with obesity. Still, there has been new evidence that Sleep Apnea can also cause it.

-**Diabetes:** In Sleep Apnea, blood sugar levels can also be disturbed due to several hormonal changes because of the brain's activity. These changes somehow can increase the risk of diabetes Type 2 in the patients. And if someone is also obese, the risk of developing Type 2 diabetes along with Sleep Apnea increases.

# Chapter 18: Importance Of Sleep

The importance of sleep can never be overestimated. In recent studies on sleeping patterns, it was revealed that a very large percentage of the population suffers from sleep deprivation. We are sleeping for less hours as other commitments take up more of our time. We are always scrambling to create more time to meet our endless demands and the only solution seems to be cutting down on the hours we sleep. It's not uncommon to hear of people sleeping for three or four hours so that they can have more time to meet deadlines. In any case, who can afford to spend so much time sleeping? In reality, we can't afford not to sleep. Sleep is very crucial in everything we do as humans. In fact, we humans are the only mammals who control our sleeping patterns to suite our liking or lifestyle. Other mammals will sleep when they are tired, but due to how busy we are as humans we ignore our biological clock so we can meet society's pressures and demands. I want us to appreciate the importance of sleep in this chapter before we get to the tips and tricks to a better night's sleep.

According to sleep experts, the first signs that we are not having enough sleep are moodiness, irritability and disinhibition. These are just the shorter term effects. Long term, chronic health problems are likely to affect us due to lack of sleep.

Sleep plays a very vital role in our wellbeing and good health. Our mental health, physical health, quality of life and safety in the workplace are all connected with the amount and quality of sleep we have. In children, sleep helps in growth and development and it is very critical that all children get a good night's sleep. The way we feel ourselves during the day is largely related to how well we slept or vice versa. I am sure you have felt moody, emotional or just plain bored during the day after having a disturbed sleep. This is because sleep supports the brain function which controls everything we do. Let's look at the importance of sleep in greater detail

Emotional wellbeing and healthy brain function

When we sleep, our brains are still working, they are preparing for the next day. The brain uses the time spent sleeping clearing most of the information we had accumulated during the day from our temporary memory too more permanent memory. Thus clearing the way for more pathways that will help you be prepared for the next day. This shows the importance of sleep in learning and memory. This is not only important to those in school but everyone of us since we are constantly learning new things each day. Sleep also improves our brains capacity to solve problems and find appropriate solutions.

Sleep deficiency alters the function of the brain, leading to a poor control of our emotions, trouble in making decisions and coping with even the slightest changes to our normal schedules. In a recent studies, sleep deprivation has also been linked with depression, suicide and risky behavior.

Physical health

We need sleep to keep our bodies in their optimal physical shape. One issue that the world is grappling with right now is obesity. There have been numerous studies researching on the link between sleeping patterns and obesity. In almost all of them, the results have shown that sleep deficiency increases the risk of obesity greatly. One explanation advanced towards this is that sleep maintains a good balance of the hormones which makes us feel hungry or full. Sleep also controls the levels of insulin in our system. Insulin regulates the amount of sugar in our blood. When we don't get enough sleep, the hunger hormones increase leading to more binge eating during the day. Other chronic health problems such as heart disease, kidney disease, high blood pressure, stroke and diabetes have a connection with poor sleep. When we sleep, the body repairs our damaged tissues and restores the balance in the functioning of the body organs. Our heart and blood vessels need sleep to repair and heal them since they are constantly working hard to circulate blood.

Our immune system heavily relies on sleep to work properly. Our immune system protects us against any infections, viruses and harmful substances. When we don't get enough sleep, we are more susceptible to common infections and illnesses.

Performance and safety

Sleep is extremely important in how we perform our day to day activities. When you don't sleep well, you are less productive and susceptible to making mistakes at work or school. You may also endanger yourself and others if operating in a high risk environment. This is what happens, when we don't get enough sleep, we are likely to have micro sleep. These are short episodes of sleep while we are still awake. This is normally what happens when you see someone dozing off unintentionally. This greatly affects our performance. In case we are operating heavy machinery or driving, we endanger ourselves and those close to us. We are not in control of micro sleep however much we might try to keep alert. In fact if you ever find yourself dozing off or not remembering what you had done shortly earlier, then the best solution would be to take some time off and have a nap.

Sleep is not just some time we lie in bed and shut off. It's a time when our body takes the opportunity to do some massive repair and restoration. It's akin to the regular service equipment's needs. Do a 'shoddy' service and you'll be in line for a huge breakdown. We have seen some of the critical functions that go on when we sleep. In order to be in top condition and work at full potential, we need not to reduce the amount of hours we sleep but to add them. An average adult will need 7-9 hours of sleep each day. Having enough sleep is extremely important to us. It's not just the amount of hours we sleep but also the quality of sleep. Sleep is a process we go through. Right from the time we go to bed to when we wake up; our body will have gone through several distinct stages of sleep. With each stage, different physiological processes will take place. These stages build and go through cycles throughout the night. You are not in control of these stages and any interruption at any stage will have some effects on you. Your role here is setting aside adequate time to facilitate a good night's sleep. This is what we call quality of sleep. There are several tips and trick to ensure this and we'll be discussing them in the subsequent chapters.

# Conclusion

With these life hacks and strategies in place, you will find that your nightly rest is becoming a natural part of your routine. Instead of lying awake, your mind restlessly reviewing the events of the day and its challenges, you will be drifting off to sleep with ease.

Because of your newly enhanced sleep life, lived out in your dedicated sanctuary, you will be waking up feeling more refreshed and rested; ready to take on the day.

Your new life habits, having become intimate friends and supports, are leading you to better health, productivity and the kind of positive attitude that people respond to. That means a better life for you, lived more fully.

Don't be surprised if people look at you and tell you that you look rested, refreshed and maybe even younger!

Because you've taken control of your life and taken back your time, you're now feeling better than you've felt in a very long time.

The power of a good night's sleep is now yours. Sleep well, my friends! Feel amazing!

Ingram Content Group UK Ltd.
Milton Keynes UK
UKHW021135230323
419044UK00015B/464

9 781990 268359